Thriving With Parkinson's Disease

Perspectives And Strategies For A Fulfilling Life

Dr. John I. Hedley Ph.D

Dedication

This Book Represents Our Common Journey Of Self Discovery And Resilience To Everyone Dealing With Parkinson's. May It Guide You Into Empowerment..

Table of Contents

Writers Review

This book, which sets out on a literary voyage to navigate the rough seas of Parkinson's disease, proves to be a beacon of hope for everyone trying to make their way through the complexity of this neurological disorder. The author creates a story that is both educational and encouraging, speaking with a voice that is both competent and well acquainted with the difficulties experienced by patients and their caretakers.

With careful attention to detail, the table of contents offers each chapter as a stepping stone through the disease's evolution, providing insights into the medical, psychological, and societal issues that it brings. The writer's skill in simplifying intricate medical ideas into comprehensible and realistic content serves as a guiding light for readers who would be lost in a sea of doubt.

It is my honer as a writer's reviewer to praise the author for their commitment to raising awareness about Parkinson's disease. Their dedication to informing and empowering individuals impacted by the illness is demonstrated by this book. It is an invaluable tool that should inspire, encourage, and lead.

Introduction

Have you ever wondered what it might be like to be powerless over your own body? To feel your hands shake uncontrollably, your muscles stiffen, and your speech become slurred? to find it hard to do everyday tasks like dressing, eating, and walking? To risk losing consciousness, sinking into memory, and experiencing depression? This is the daily reality for millions of people across the world who suffer with Parkinson's disease, a degenerative neurological illness that affects movement and other aspects of health.

Parkinson's disease is a condition in which parts of the brain become damaged over time. This leads to a shortage of a chemical called dopamine, which helps the brain control the body's movements. Without enough dopamine, people with Parkinson's disease have problems with coordination, balance, and speed. They also experience other symptoms, such as mood changes, sleep problems, pain, and cognitive impairment.

Although the precise origin of Parkinson's disease is unknown, a mix of environmental and hereditary factors is thought to be involved. While some people may be exposed to chemicals or diseases that cause the condition, others may inherit a higher chance of contracting it. Parkinson's disease primarily affects the elderly, however it can strike anybody at any age. It affects men somewhat more frequently than it does women. The World Health Organisation estimates that approximately 8.5 million individuals worldwide suffer with Parkinson's disease, and as the population ages, this figure is projected to rise.

This book aims to provide readers a thorough and approachable overview of Parkinson's disease, covering everything from diagnosis and treatment to effects on everyday functioning and overall quality of life. This book is meant for anybody who is interested in learning more about this illness, regardless of whether they are merely inquisitive or have knowledge of someone who has it. As a neurologist with over 20 years of experience, I have seen firsthand how Parkinson's affects patients as well as my own family members. By imparting my knowledge and experience, I want to be able to better comprehend and manage this difficult illness.

You will discover more about Parkinson's disease symptoms, causes, diagnosis, and therapy in the upcoming chapters. Along with learning how to get resources and assistance, you will also learn how to handle the psychological, emotional, and physical elements of having the condition. With this book, I wish to provide you with more knowledge on Parkinson's disease and provide you the tools you need to take control of your well-being. I appreciate you reading, and if you have any questions or comments, don't hesitate to get in touch with me. Never forget that there is always hope and that you are not alone on this road.

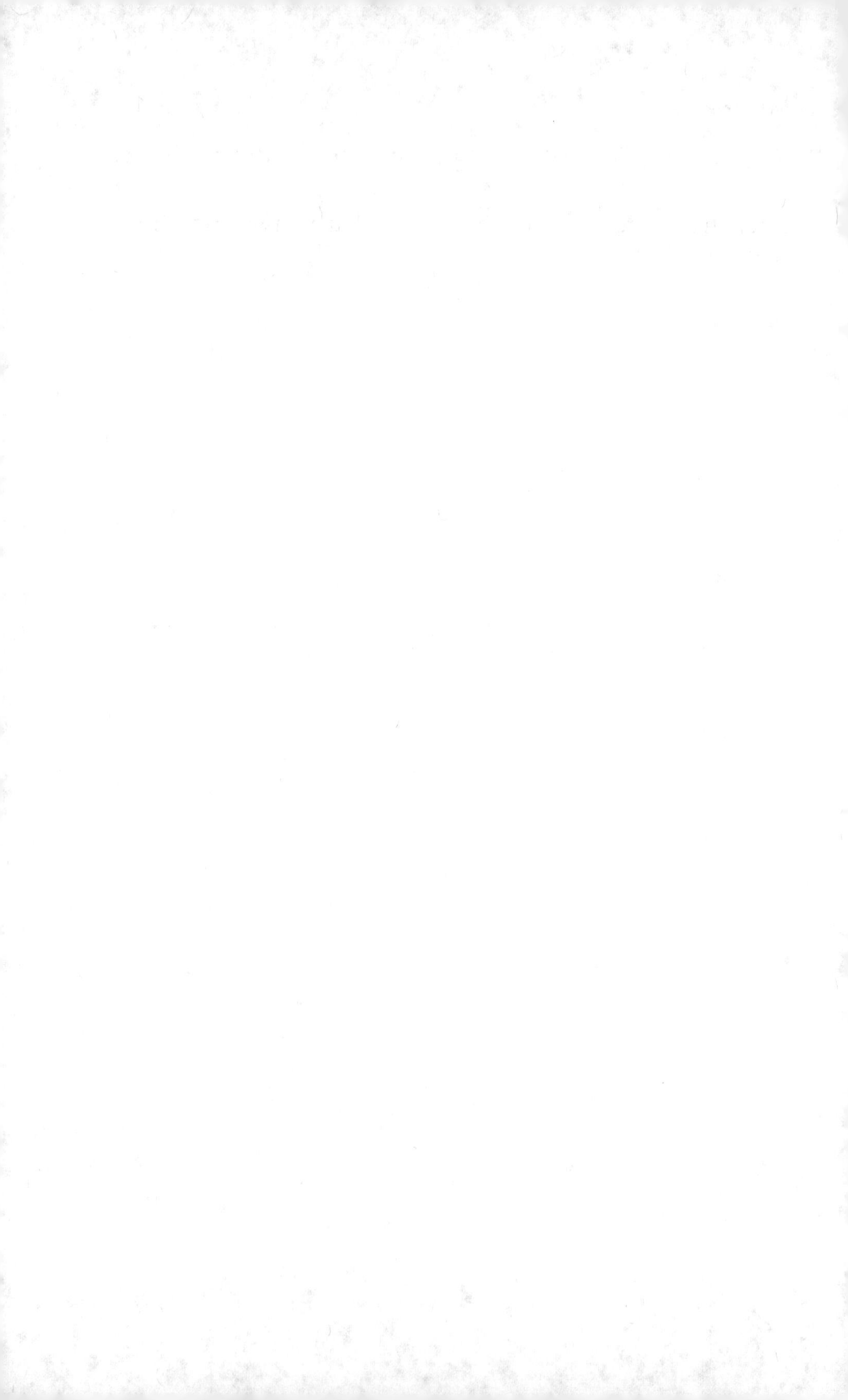

Chapter One

UNDERSTANDING PARKINSON'S DISEASE

Parkinson's disease is a neurological condition that impairs sensation and movement. It results from the death or malfunction of some of the brain cells that produce the neurotransmitter dopamine. Dopamine functions as a messenger to instruct your muscles. Your motions become harder, stiffer, and slower as your dopamine levels drop. Additionally, you can experience issues with your posture, balance, and coordination. Daily tasks like eating, talking, walking, and dressing may become more difficult and stressful as a result.

However, Parkinson's disease affects more than only mobility. It may also have an impact on other areas of your health and wellbeing, including your digestion, mood, memory, sleep, and level of pain. Depression, anxiety, dementia, or hallucinations can affect certain people. Others could experience difficulties with swallowing, sleeping, or managing their bowels or bladder. Individual differences may exist in these symptoms, and they could evolve over time.

Although the precise causation of Parkinson's disease is unknown, a number of variables most likely contribute to it. A portion of these variables are inherited from your parents, or genetic in nature. Others are environmental, which means they have to do with things like diseases, poisons, or brain trauma. Certain individuals may be more susceptible to Parkinson's disease due to factors such as age, gender, or ethnicity. For instance, men, older individuals, and those with European ancestry are more likely to get Parkinson's disease.

The symptoms of Parkinson's disease cannot be cured, but there are therapies that can help you live a better, more comfortable life. Medication is the most popular kind of therapy as it can help your brain's dopamine levels return and lessen some of your mobility issues. Medication comes in a variety of forms, and each might have unique effects and negative effects. Your physician will assist you in selecting the appropriate medicine and adjusting the dosage as necessary.

Surgery is an additional therapy option that entails implanting a device in your brain that communicates electrical impulses to the regions responsible for controlling movement. This may lessen some of the Parkinson's disease-related tremors, stiffness, and slowness. Surgery carries certain risks and problems, so it's not appropriate for everyone. Your physician will discuss the advantages and disadvantages of surgery with you and assist you in making an informed decision.

Physical therapy, occupational therapy, speech therapy, and psychological therapy are further forms of treatment. These can support your emotional well-being, function, mobility, and communication. They can also provide you with coping mechanisms, tactics, and exercise regimens to help you manage your disease. Complementary therapies like yoga, meditation, acupuncture, and massage may potentially be beneficial to you. These can ease your tension, promote relaxation, and enhance your general wellbeing.

The most crucial thing to keep in mind is that you are not travelling alone. You have a lot of individuals in your life that can relate to, support, and understand you. These include of medical professionals such as physicians, nurses, therapists, and other family members and friends. Another option is to sign up for a support group, where you may converse with others who have Parkinson's disease, exchange stories, and gain knowledge from one another. Organisations that focus on Parkinson's disease, including the Parkinson's Foundation, the Michael J. Fox Foundation, or the World Parkinson Coalition, can also provide you with resources, information, and guidance.

Although it might be difficult, Parkinson's illness does not define you. You may still pursue your own objectives and follow your hobbies and yet lead a happy and meaningful life. You can continue to appreciate your favourite things and find new ones to like. With your bravery and tenacity, you can still change the world and motivate others. You are still who you are.

Chapter Two

COPING WITH THE DIAGNOSIS

Finding out you have Parkinson's disease may be a devastating and life-altering event. You can be filled with a lot of uncertainties, worries, and feelings. You could be concerned about how Parkinson's disease will impact your life, relationships, health, and future. You could feel furious, perplexed, or alone. You could also experience optimism, relief, or hope. When someone is told they have Parkinson's disease, there is no right or incorrect way to feel or respond. Everybody has a distinct and diverse experience.

It is not impossible to deal with a Parkinson's disease diagnosis, though. Parkinson's disease can be effectively managed if you can learn to accept, comprehend, and live with your illness.

Understanding the process of diagnosis and medical assessments

The diagnosis of Parkinson's disease can be a difficult and drawn-out procedure. Parkinson's disease cannot be ruled out or confirmed by a single test or scan. Rather, the diagnosis is made using a number of variables, including:

- Your symptoms and medical history

- A neurological and physical assessment

- Reaction to pharmacological trial

- Extra examinations and scans, such DAT, MRI, CT, PET, or blood tests

Several healthcare providers, including the following, may be involved in

the diagnostic and medical evaluation process:

- A primary care physician qualified to offer both general care and recommendations

- A neurologist with expertise in nerve system and brain issues

- A specialist in movement disorders with potential knowledge of Parkinson's disease and other movement problems

- A neuropsychologist who can evaluate your emotional and cognitive abilities

- A speech-language pathologist who can assess and manage your swallowing and speech issues.

- An occupational therapist who can support you with everyday tasks and independence; a physical therapist who can aid with balance, mobility, and exercise.

- A social worker who may offer you services, information, and assistance

Individual differences may exist in the diagnostic and medical evaluation procedure based on your needs, condition, and symptoms. Receiving a conclusive diagnosis of Parkinson's disease may take months or years. It may also alter over time due to changes in your health and symptoms. As a result, it's critical to schedule routine check-ups and follow-ups with your medical team and to be transparent and honest with them about any changes or worries you may have.

Interpreting your test results and what they mean

You may have tests and scans that are necessary for the diagnosis and medical evaluations, and these procedures might yield important details about your health and condition. They may, however, also be perplexing and challenging to understand. You might be curious about the significance of your test findings and how they connect to your Parkinson's disease diagnosis. The following advice and recommendations will help you understand the meaning of your test results:

Make inquiries and look for explanation. Asking questions and getting clarification from your healthcare staff on the meaning of your test findings shouldn't be seen as shameful or awkward. They are there to elucidate and assist you in understanding your health and condition. "What does this test measure?" one may wonder, for example. Which ranges are typical and abnormal? What ramifications and potential causes may my test findings have? How do the findings of my tests impact my diagnosis and course of care? How many times must I take this test again?

Conduct independent research. You may also conduct independent research to find out more about the possible tests and scans you may have and what they entail. You may utilise trustworthy and authoritative information sources, such books, articles, websites, and online platforms, to learn about Parkinson's disease and its diagnosis and medical evaluations. But, you should always double-check the information you obtain with your medical team and use caution and scepticism. Additionally, as self-diagnosis and self-treatment based on test findings can be hazardous and detrimental, you should refrain from doing so.

Maintain a log and monitor your test findings. You may also maintain a log and monitor the evolution of your test findings over time. A notepad, a spreadsheet, a mobile application, or any other tool that suits your needs can be used. Information like the test's date, time, name, type, result, and interpretation can all be tracked and recorded. You can also record the medication you were taking at the time of the test, its dosage, any symptoms or side effects you experienced before, during, or after the test, and any questions or comments you may have about the test. You may have a better overview and comprehension of your health and condition by maintaining a record of your test findings and monitoring them. Additionally, you can address any changes or worries you may have with your healthcare provider after sharing your test findings with them.

Addressing your emotions and concerns after receiving a diagnosis

Finding out you have Parkinson's disease might cause a variety of feelings and worries. Shock, incredulity, denial, rage, anguish, grief, fear, worry, guilt, humiliation, or melancholy are possible emotions. In addition, you could experience appreciation, acceptance, hope, optimism, relief, or empowerment. It's possible for you to feel many emotions at various moments, or even simultaneously. Other worries you can have include: What impact will Parkinson's disease have on my relationships, future, health, and quality of life? How will I handle Parkinson's disease symptoms and obstacles? Which available treatments are appropriate for me? How am I going to cover Parkinson's disease bills and expenses? Where can I get Parkinson's disease support and assistance?

After learning of your diagnosis, it might be difficult but not impossible to deal with your feelings and worries. With Parkinson's disease, you may learn to manage your feelings and anxieties and have a fulfilling life. Following a diagnosis, the following advice and recommendations might help you deal with your feelings and worries:

Express and acknowledge your feelings and worries. Your feelings and worries may worsen if you ignore or repress them, which might have an adverse effect on your health and general wellbeing. Rather, accept and communicate your feelings and worries, and then let them out. There are several methods you might communicate your feelings and worries, such speaking with a trusted family member, friend, medical expert, or therapist. writing a letter, a poem, a blog, or a journal. Painting, drawing, or producing anything. Performing music, dancing, or singing. praying, meditating, or engaging in mindfulness exercises. engaging in a pleasurable and soothing activity, like playing, watching, or reading.

Ask for and accept support and assistance from others. It's not necessary for you to handle your feelings and worries by yourself. It is possible to ask for and receive assistance and support from others who can relate to you and provide you with direction, counsel, consolation, or aid. These might be anybody who can support you in managing your emotions and worries, such as your therapist, coach, support group, friends, family, or medical team. You may lessen your feelings of stress and loneliness and boost your self-esteem and motivation by asking for and receiving assistance and support from others. In addition, you'll feel more understood and supported as you develop and fortify your bonds with other people.

Take time to familiarise yourself with Parkinson's disease. Studying and educating yourself on Parkinson's disease might also help you manage your feelings and worries. You may utilise trustworthy and legitimate information sources, such books, articles, websites, and online platforms, to learn about Parkinson's disease and its symptoms, causes, diagnosis, therapy, and management.

These sources offer credible and thorough information. Additionally, you may go to conferences, workshops, webinars, seminars, and other events where leaders and specialists in the field of Parkinson's disease are featured. You can obtain understanding and perspective about your health and circumstances by being knowledgeable about Parkinson's disease. You may also be aware of your alternatives and choices so that you can make wise judgements with confidence. Not only can you defeat stigma and prejudice, but you can also debunk myths and preconceptions.

Chapter Three

MANAGING THE SYMPTOMS OF PARKINSON'S DISEASE

There are many different symptoms of Parkinson's disease that can impact your mobility, happiness, and general well-being. These signs and symptoms might differ from person to person and evolve over time. Among the most typical symptoms are:

- Tremor: A trembling or swaying of the hands, arms, legs, jaw, or face, often during repose or relaxation.

- Rigidity: A tautness or rigidity of muscles, particularly in the trunk, arms, and legs.

- Bradykinesia is the inability or slowness to initiate or maintain motor functions including walking, turning, or reaching.

- A lack of balance or a propensity to tumble, particularly while shifting postures or directions, is known as postural instability.

- Depression is characterised by a lingering sense of hopelessness, unhappiness, or disinterest in activities you used to like.

- Anxiety is a state of unease, concern, or terror that obstructs day-to-day functioning.

- Cognitive impairment refers to issues with thinking, planning, memory, or solving difficulties.

- Difficulties in falling, staying, or waking up from sleep. Moreover, you can experience nightmares, sleep talking, or vivid dreams.

- Pain is a feeling of pain or hurting in the joints, muscles, or nerves. In addition, you can get cramps, headaches, or restless legs.

- Constipation is defined as having fewer bowel motions than normal or having trouble passing faeces.

- Urinary issues include feeling the need to urinate more frequently or urgently, as well as having trouble initiating or halting the flow of urine.

- Reduced libido, trouble obtaining or keeping an erection, and trouble experiencing an orgasm are examples of sexual issues.

Your relationships, self-esteem, and overall quality of life may all be impacted by these symptoms. They may also make it more difficult for you to pursue your needs and desires, such working, learning, socialising, or engaging in your hobbies.

How to treat your symptoms with medication, surgery, or other therapies

The symptoms of Parkinson's disease cannot be cured, but there are therapies that can help you manage them and enhance your quality of life. Medication is the most popular kind of therapy as it can help your brain's dopamine levels return and lessen some of your mobility issues. Medication comes in a variety of forms, and each might have unique effects and negative effects. Your physician will assist you in selecting the appropriate medicine and adjusting the dosage as necessary.

Several of the most widely used drugs for Parkinson's disease include:

1. One medication that easily enters the brain and transforms into dopamine is levodopa. Although it

can also result in nausea, sleepiness, or uncontrollable movements (dyskinesia), it is helpful for tremor, stiffness, and bradykinesia.

2. Medications known as dopamine agonists stimulate dopamine receptors and replicate the effects of dopamine. They can be used to treat bradykinesia, stiffness, and tremor either on their own or in combination with levodopa. They may, however, also result in nausea, sleepiness, hallucinations, or problems with impulse control (such obsessive gambling or shopping).

3. MAO-B inhibitors are medications that block the action of an enzyme that breaks down dopamine, therefore increasing the quantity of dopamine in the brain. They can be used to treat bradykinesia, stiffness, and tremor either on their own or in combination with levodopa. Additionally, they may

have a little antidepressant effect. But they can also result in headaches, nausea, or sleeplessness.

4. COMT inhibitors are medications that stop another enzyme from breaking down dopamine. They have the potential to prolong the duration and efficacy of levodopa when administered in conjunction with it. But they can also result in dyskinesia, diarrhoea, or nausea.

There are more kinds of Parkinson's disease medications, but these are some of the more common ones. Other medications may be prescribed by your doctor to treat certain symptoms including pain, sadness, anxiety, insomnia, or constipation. For further medical issues including diabetes, heart disease, or high blood pressure, you might also need to take more drugs.

It's critical that you take your medicine as directed by your physician and pay close attention to their advice. Any other drugs, vitamins, or herbal treatments you take should be disclosed to your doctor as well, since they can interfere with the medicine you take for Parkinson's disease. Any adverse effects you encounter should be reported to your doctor as well, as they might be able to modify your prescription or dose to help you feel better.

Although medication can help you manage your symptoms, Parkinson's disease cannot be cured by it. Your drug may lose its effectiveness over time, or you may require greater dosages to get the same effects. This is due to the fact that your dopamine levels are continuously declining and your brain cells are still degenerating. For this reason, further therapies or surgeries could be necessary to help you manage the illness.

Surgery is an additional therapy option that entails implanting a device in your brain that communicates electrical impulses to the regions responsible for controlling movement. This may lessen some of the Parkinson's disease-related tremors, stiffness, and slowness. Surgery carries certain risks and problems, so it's not appropriate for everyone. Your physician will discuss the advantages and disadvantages of surgery with you and assist you in making an informed decision.

Physical therapy, occupational therapy, speech therapy, and psychological therapy are further forms of treatment. These can support your emotional well-being, function, mobility, and communication. They can also provide you with coping mechanisms, tactics, and exercise regimens to help you manage your disease. Complementary therapies like yoga, meditation, acupuncture, and massage may potentially be beneficial to you. These can ease your tension, promote relaxation, and enhance your general

wellbeing.

Chapter Four

TREATMENT OPTIONS FOR PARKINSON'S DISEASE

The disorder known as Parkinson's disease impairs both your motor and cognitive abilities. It results from the death or malfunction of some of the brain cells that produce the neurotransmitter dopamine. Your brain uses dopamine to regulate both your emotions and your muscles. Reduced dopamine levels can cause issues with mood, balance, stiffness, slowness, and tremors.

The symptoms of Parkinson's disease cannot be cured, but there are therapies that can help you manage them and enhance your quality of life. Medication, surgery, and further therapy are some of these treatments.

What are the non-pharmacological treatments, such as physical therapy and speech therapy?

Parkinson's disease can be treated with more than just medication. Other therapies may also be able to improve your well-being, function, mobility, and communication. Physical therapy, occupational therapy, speech therapy, and psychiatric treatment are some of these therapies. Depending on your symptoms and requirements, you could require one or more of these therapies.

Enhancing your strength, flexibility, balance, and coordination may be achieved with the use of physical therapy. It can also assist with pain management, posture maintenance, and fall prevention. You may enhance your movement and fitness by learning stretches, exercises, and other methods from a physical therapist. If you want assistance, they may also provide you advice on how to operate wheelchairs, walkers, and canes.

You can carry out your everyday tasks, like eating, working, taking a shower, and dressing, with the assistance of occupational therapy. It can also assist you in adjusting to your surroundings, including your house, place of employment, and neighbourhood. You can learn techniques, abilities, and advice from an occupational therapist to improve your quality of life and ease of living. They can also provide recommendations for equipment, tools, or adjustments to make your duties easier.

Your voice, speaking, and swallowing can all be improved with speech therapy. It can also facilitate improved cognitive and emotion expression and interpersonal communication. You may increase the clarity, loudness, and quality of your voice with the help of a speech therapist.

They can also assist you with controlling your salivary flow, coughing, and breathing. If necessary, they can also instruct you on how to utilise augmentative or alternative communication equipment, such tablets, keyboards, and applications.

You can manage the psychological and emotional elements of having Parkinson's disease with the support of psychological treatment. Additionally, it can enhance your quality of life, happiness, and sense of self. A mental health professional may provide you advice, direction, and support. Additionally, they might instruct you in coping mechanisms like mindfulness, relaxation, or cognitive-behavioural therapy. They may also assist you in resolving any problems you may be facing, like stress, bereavement, anxiety, and despair.

There are more non-pharmacological therapies for Parkinson's disease, but these are some of the more common ones. Complementary therapies like yoga, meditation, acupuncture, and massage may potentially be beneficial to you. These can ease your tension, promote relaxation, and enhance your general wellbeing. Participating in social activities like volunteering, joining a hobby club, or support groups may also be beneficial. These can facilitate social interaction, enjoyment, and the search for meaning and purpose in life.

To identify the best course of therapy for you, it's critical to collaborate with your therapist, doctor, and support system. Additionally, you ought to take charge of your own treatment and be proactive. It is important that you adhere to your treatment plan and let your doctor or therapist know about any changes or issues. Additionally, you ought to ask for assistance when required and don't be afraid to voice your worries or pose inquiries. You have the right to take an active role in your own treatment since you are the expert on your own experience.

Although treatment can help you manage your symptoms, Parkinson's disease cannot be cured. Your condition could vary over time, necessitating modifications

to your treatment plan. For this reason, it could be necessary

for you to stay up to date on the most recent advancements

and studies related to Parkinson's disease.

What are the emerging therapies and research advancements?

As a complicated and difficult disorder, Parkinson's disease still has a lot of unanswered questions. Researchers and scientists are always trying to come up with fresh and improved approaches to comprehend, manage, and even cure the illness. Among the cutting-edge treatments and scientific discoveries are:

Gene therapy is a procedure whereby genes are altered or inserted into brain cells to improve or rectify their function. This may lessen the risk of brain injury, enhance dopamine synthesis, or alter the function of other brain chemicals. Gene therapy has various hazards and limits and is still in the experimental stage of development. In human studies and animal models, it has, nonetheless, demonstrated some encouraging outcomes.

Stem cell treatment is a procedure that replaces or repairs damaged brain cells using stem cells, which are cells with the ability to differentiate into multiple types of cells. This may lessen mobility issues, raise dopamine levels, and stop the illness from becoming worse. Additionally, stem cell treatment is still in its experimental phase and presents some technological, legal, and ethical difficulties. Nonetheless, research on humans and animal models has indicated some possible advantages.

Utilising the body's own immune system to combat the illness is known as immunotherapy. This may aid in lowering inflammation, removing harmful proteins, or promoting the development of new brain cells. Additionally yet at the experimental stage, immunotherapy comes with potential risks and adverse effects. Nonetheless, studies on humans and animal models have revealed some beneficial benefits.

Medications known as neuroprotective medicines can shield brain cells from further harm or degeneration. This can assist maintain the residual dopamine levels while slowing or stopping the disease's development. Research on neuroprotective drugs is ongoing, and their efficacy and safety have not yet been shown. However, in experiments conducted on humans and animal models, they have produced some encouraging outcomes.

There are more new treatments and scientific developments for Parkinson's disease in addition to these. New findings and advancements in the field of Parkinson's disease are being discovered on a daily basis. By following reliable sites like the Parkinson's Foundation, the Michael J.

Fox Foundation, or the World Parkinson Coalition, you may stay up to date on the most recent news and advancements. Clinical trials, which are investigations testing novel therapies or approaches for Parkinson's disease, offer another option for participation. Clinical trials have the potential to expand scientific understanding and enhance Parkinson's disease patient treatment. Speak with your doctor or browse websites like ClinicalTrials.gov (https://clinicaltrials.gov/) or Fox Trial Finder (https://foxtrialfinder.michaeljfox.org/) to learn more about clinical trials and how to enrol in them.

Although treatment can help you manage your symptoms, Parkinson's disease cannot be cured. Nonetheless, there is hope for the future since scientists and researchers are putting a lot of effort into coming up with fresh approaches to comprehend, manage, and perhaps cure the illness. You can contribute to this hope by continuing to be knowledgeable, engaged, and positive. By sharing your voice, experience, and narrative with other Parkinson's disease sufferers, you too can contribute to this hope. With your bravery and tenacity, you have the power to inspire people and change the world.

Chapter Five

LIVING WELL WITH PARKINSON'S DISEASE

The disorder known as Parkinson's disease impairs both your motor and cognitive abilities. It results from the death or malfunction of some of the brain cells that produce the neurotransmitter dopamine. Your brain uses dopamine to regulate both your emotions and your muscles. Reduced dopamine levels can cause issues with mood, balance, stiffness, slowness, and tremors.

The effects of Parkinson's disease can be profound on your life, relationships, and general wellbeing. It may make it more difficult for you to pursue your needs and desires, including working, learning, socialising, and engaging in your hobbies. It may also have an impact on your enjoyment, confidence, and sense of self. Nonetheless, there are methods for managing Parkinson's disease properly. Having your own objectives, aspirations, and hobbies does not exclude you from leading a happy and meaningful life. You can continue to appreciate your favourite things and find new ones to like. With your bravery and tenacity, you can still change the world and motivate others.

How to maintain your quality of life after a diagnosis

Receiving a Parkinson's disease diagnosis might come as a shock. You can experience fear, rage, sadness, or confusion. How this will impact your life, your family, and your future may be on your mind. You might not know where to look for assistance and you could have a lot of questions and worries. These are typical responses, and you're not the only one who experiences them.

First of all, there is no guarantee that someone with Parkinson's disease will die. Being a chronic and progressive illness, it does not kill you; instead, it deteriorates over time. You may enhance your quality of life and control your symptoms with the aid of some therapies. The psychological and practical difficulties of having the illness can also be managed. You may still pursue your own objectives and follow your hobbies and yet lead a happy and meaningful life.

Second, each person's experience with Parkinson's disease is unique. Individual differences exist in the symptoms, course, and responsiveness to therapy. The condition cannot be treated with a one-size-fits-all strategy. You need to be adaptable and willing to modify while figuring out what works best for you. You must also take the initiative and participate in your own treatment. To identify the greatest answers for your requirements, you must collaborate with your therapist, doctor, and support system.

Thirdly, realise that you are not traveling alone on this adventure. You have a lot of individuals in your life that can relate to, support, and understand you. These include of medical professionals such as physicians, nurses, therapists, and other family members and friends. Another option is to sign up for a support group, where you may converse with others who have Parkinson's disease, exchange stories, and gain knowledge from one another. Organisations that focus on Parkinson's disease, such the World Parkinson Coalition, the Michael J. Fox Foundation, and the Parkinson's Foundation, can also provide you with resources, information, and guidance.

Following a diagnosis, there are three things you must do to preserve your quality of life: accept, adjust, and act.

Accept: Giving up or losing hope does not entail accepting your diagnosis. It entails accepting the truth of your circumstances and being aware of your advantages and disadvantages. It entails communicating your wants and feelings and being truthful with both yourself and other people. It implies not blaming yourself or anybody else for your situation and practicing self-compassion. You may be able to manage your stress, worry, and sadness better if you accept your diagnosis. It may also assist you in appreciating what you have and your abilities and helping you concentrate on the good parts of your life.

Adapt: Changing your expectations, surroundings, and way of life will help you adjust to your diagnosis. It entails being inventive and adaptable and coming up with new ways to accomplish the tasks you need to or want to complete. It entails employing tools, equipment, or assistance technologies to help you do your job. It entails accepting assistance when it is given and asking for aid when you need it. It entails defining reasonable, attainable objectives and acknowledging your successes. You can get through whatever obstacles you may encounter by learning to live with your condition. Additionally, it can support you in preserving your dignity, independence, and capacity.

Act: Taking steps to enhance your happiness, well-being, and health is a crucial part of acting on your diagnosis. It entails adhering to your specified course of care and taking your prescription on time. It entails consistent exercise, a healthy diet, and restful sleep. It include discovering new interests or hobbies as well as partaking in enjoyable activities. It entails making new acquaintances and maintaining relationships with loved ones. It entails taking involved in voluntary work, advocacy, or research. Taking action after receiving a diagnosis can assist you in controlling your symptoms, avoiding complications, and slowing the disease's course. You can make a difference in the world and discover meaning and purpose in your life with its assistance.

You may live well with Parkinson's disease and preserve your quality of life by acknowledging, adjusting to, and acting upon your diagnosis. By your bravery and tenacity, you may encourage people and demonstrate to them that having Parkinson's disease does not define you. You remain who you are.

How to manage your daily activities and adapt to changes

It may be more difficult to accomplish the activities you need or want to do, including work, study, socialise, or engage in hobbies, if you have Parkinson's disease. It may also result in adjustments to your requirements, preferences, and talents. Your everyday routines, like eating, dressing, taking a shower, and driving, may be impacted by these changes. You can control your everyday activities and adjust to changes, though. You can discover new avenues for enjoyment in life and continue to do many of the activities you like.

Three skills are necessary to effectively manage daily tasks and adjust to changes: planning, prioritising, and pacing.

Plan: You may better manage your time, energy, and resources by creating a plan for your everyday tasks. It can also assist you in becoming ready for any obstacles or problems you could encounter. To organise your day, week, or month, you can use an app, a planner, a notebook, or a calendar. To assist you in remembering your responsibilities and appointments, you may also utilise timers, alarms, and reminders. Your activities should be scheduled in accordance with your mood, your medication, and your symptoms. For example, when your medicine is functioning well and you are feeling alert and energised, you might want to focus on the most critical or challenging activities. When your symptoms are at their worst or when you're feeling anxious or exhausted, you might also wish to refrain from performing specific jobs. In order to keep your energy levels up and avoid being exhausted, you need schedule in some pauses, relaxation, and rest throughout the day.

Set priorities: Setting priorities for your daily tasks can help you concentrate on the things that are most essential to you and let go of the things that are superfluous or unimportant. You may feel less guilty, frustrated, and stressed as a result of it. To rank your tasks according to priority and urgency, you can use a matrix, chart, or list. You may also evaluate your activities according to your level of interest and enjoyment by using a rating system, such a scale from 1 to 10. Activities should be prioritised based on your beliefs, objectives, and personal preferences. For instance, you could wish to focus on activities that are important to you or that are necessary, like looking after your family, your career, or your health. You could also wish to pursue your interests, your hobbies, or your dreams—things that bring you joy or satisfaction. Certain tasks, like doing housework, doing errands, or going to events, may be less important to you and should be delegated, put off, or eliminated.

Pace: You may balance your workload, rest, and pleasure by keeping a regular schedule for your everyday tasks. It can also assist you in avoiding the boom-and-bust cycle and not overdoing or under-doing your tasks. You may pace your activities according to your demands, your restrictions, and your talents by using a clock, a stopwatch, or a timer. You may also keep an eye on your activities, symptoms, and emotions by keeping a journal, log, or tracker. Your energy, endurance, and comfort levels should all be taken into consideration while pacing your activities. For instance, instead of working on your tasks over extended periods of time with little pauses, you might wish to perform them in short bursts. Rather than engaging in one activity for an extended period of time, you could also want to switch up your routine by undertaking several kinds of activities, such mental, social, or physical ones. In addition, you might wish to modify your speed based on external factors like the surrounding individuals, the time of day, or the weather.

You can manage your everyday tasks and adjust to changes by prioritizing, pacing, and planning them. Your function, performance, and enjoyment can all be enhanced. Additionally, you have the power to improve your happiness, well-being, and standard of living.

How to exercise, eat well, and sleep well

Your health and wellbeing depend on exercise, proper diet, and adequate sleep, particularly if you have Parkinson's disease. They can assist you in controlling your symptoms, avoiding problems, and slowing down the illness's course. Additionally, they can boost your confidence, vitality, and happiness. We'll provide some advice on how to work out, eat healthfully, and sleep properly in this area.

How to Work Out

If you have Parkinson's disease, getting exercise is one of the finest things you can do for yourself. Your strength, flexibility, balance, and coordination may all be enhanced by it. Additionally, it might lessen your bradykinesia, stiffness, and tremor. It can also assist with pain management, posture maintenance, and fall prevention. Additionally, exercise can enhance your mood, memory, and cognitive function. Additionally, it can aid in the reduction of anxiety, sadness, and tension.

To maximize the health advantages of physical activity, adhere to following recommendations:

Before beginning any fitness regimen, speak with your doctor. Your doctor may offer you advice on how to exercise safely and successfully as well as assist you in selecting the best kind of exercise for you. Also, your doctor can keep an eye on your health and change your prescription as necessary.

- Pick an activity that fits your skills, interests, and abilities. Exercises like walking, cycling, swimming, dancing, yoga, tai chi, or boxing are among the options you may attempt. Additionally, you can enroll in a class, group, or program specifically intended for those with Parkinson's disease, such [Pedalling for Parkinson's Disease], [Dance for Parkinson's Disease], or [Rock Steady Boxing] (https://www.rocksteadyboxing.org/).

- At least three times a week, for a minimum of half an hour, engage in regular exercise. Exercise can also be divided into shorter periods, such ten minutes, three times a day. Exercise may also be included into regular activities like playing with your grandchildren, gardening, or climbing stairs.

- Engage in moderate-intensity exercise, meaning that while your breathing and heart rate should increase, you shouldn't become too dizzy or uneasy. To rate your perceived exertion, use a scale from 1 to 10, where 1 is extremely easy and 10 is very hard. Aim for a level of five or six, which indicates that you are exerting yourself, but not excessively.

- Before you workout, warm up, and after, cool down. You may increase your flexibility, lessen muscular pain, and avoid injuries by doing this. Gentle stretches or low-intensity exercises like cycling or walking might help you warm up. By performing additional stretches or using relaxation methods like breathing exercises or meditation, you can decompress.

Honor your boundaries and pay attention to your body. Exercise at your own speed without comparing yourself to other people. It's important to monitor your symptoms and how they impact your workout regimen. If you experience discomfort, dizziness, nausea, or shortness of breath, you should stop or reduce your speed. Resting is also advised if you are feeling exhausted, have a fever, an illness, or a flare-up of your symptoms.

You may live well with Parkinson's disease and enhance your physical, mental, and emotional well-being by engaging in regular exercise. In addition, you may socialize, make new friends, and find new interests.

How to have a healthy diet

It's critical to eat healthily for your overall wellbeing, particularly if you have Parkinson's disease. It can support the maintenance of your immune system, energy level, and weight. Additionally, it can aid in symptom management, avert problems, and slow down the disease's advancement. Additionally, it can enhance your mood, memory, and cognitive function. Additionally, it can aid in the reduction of anxiety, sadness, and tension.

In order to eat healthily, you should do the following:

- Consume items from all the dietary categories, such as fruits, vegetables, grains, dairy products, and protein, in a balanced and diverse diet. The [MyPlate] (https://www.myplate.gov/) concept can assist you in organizing your snacks and meals. Aim for half your plate to consist of fruits and vegetables, 25% to be grains, and 25% to be protein. A dish of dairy, such as cheese, yoghurt, or milk, should be included in your dinner or snack.

- Opt for meals high in fibre, antioxidants, and omega-3 fatty acids; they can lower inflammation, enhance intestinal function, and shield brain cells. Berries, leafy greens, nuts, seeds, beans, lentils, whole grains, salmon, and olive oil are a few of these foods.

- Foods heavy in fat, sugar, salt, and additives should be avoided since they can exacerbate symptoms, raise the risk of complications, and affect cognitive function. Fried meals, processed foods, fast food, sweets, cakes, pastries, soda, and alcoholic beverages are a few examples of these foods.

- Water is the best drink to consume in order to keep hydrated, avoid constipation, and remove toxins from the body. Aim for eight glasses of water or more if you exercise, perspire, or use medicine each day. You can also drink other liquids, such milk, juice, tea, coffee, or coffee, but keep your alcohol, sugar, and caffeine intake to a minimum because these substances might interfere with your medicine, sleep, and mood.

Consider your symptoms and medicines while planning the timing of your meals and snacks. Meals and snacks should be had on a regular basis; they shouldn't be skipped or put off. Large or heavy meals should also be avoided since they might cause nausea, bloating, and sluggishness. Additionally, you should know how certain foods affect the way your medications work, particularly levodopa. When levodopa is given empty-handed or at least half an hour before or after a meal, its absorption is optimal. However, taking levodopa without meals may cause nausea or upset stomach in certain individuals. If so, you might take it with a small snack like a glass of milk, a banana, or a cracker. Levodopa's absorption and efficiency may be hampered by eating high-protein meals like meat, cheese, or eggs right before or right after taking it. Protein is still allowed, but it should be consumed throughout the day, preferably in the evening when your levodopa dosage is lower.

You may live well with Parkinson's disease and enhance your physical, mental, and emotional well-being by consuming a healthy diet. Along with enjoying your meal, you may try out various flavors and cuisines.

How to get a good night's sleep

It's critical for your health and wellbeing to get enough sleep, particularly if you have Parkinson's disease. It can assist you in regaining your mental clarity, energy, and mood. Additionally, it can aid in symptom management, avert problems, and slow down the disease's advancement. Additionally, it can aid in the reduction of anxiety, sadness, and tension.

Nonetheless, if you have Parkinson's disease, getting a good night's sleep might be difficult. You can experience difficulties going to sleep, remaining asleep, or waking up. Moreover, you can experience nightmares, sleep talking, or vivid dreams. Additionally, you can have the unpleasant need to move your legs, especially at night, known as restless legs syndrome. Additionally, you can have sleep apnea, a disorder that results in breathing pauses during the night, generally known as snoring.

To have a good night's sleep, you should do the following:

- By going to bed and getting up at the same times every day, you can maintain a regular sleep schedule.

Your body's natural clock, the circadian rhythm, informs you when to sleep and when to get up. This can help you control it. Additionally, it can aid in preventing jet lag, which can exacerbate symptoms and interfere with sleep.

- Establish a calm and comfortable sleeping environment. Your bedroom should be cool, quiet, dark, and inviting. To block out any light, you can use eye masks or curtains, blinds, or shades. To drown out noise, use earplugs, a fan, or a white noise machine. You may also utilise calming noises like music, the sounds of nature, or meditation. In addition, you may utilise a fan, heater, or humidifier, as well as modify your room's ventilation, temperature, and humidity. Additionally, you may customise the comfort of your bed by using mattresses, pillows, blankets, and sheets that you like.

- Prior to retiring to bed, establish a calming routine and engage in a calming activity. You can stretch gently, meditate, pray, read a book, or listen to music. In addition, you can massage your feet, have a cup of herbal tea, or take a warm bath. Anything that makes you feel agitated or stressed out should be avoided, including watching TV, using a computer, phone, or tablet, working, studying, or getting into arguments. In addition, you should abstain from alcohol, cigarettes, and caffeine as these substances might cause sleep disturbances or keep you awake.

- Adhere to your doctor's directions regarding the dosage of your medicine and take it as directed. Certain drugs have the potential to improve your quality of sleep, while others may cause disruptions. To maximise the amount and quality of your sleep, your doctor can assist you in modifying the dosage or timing of your prescription. If you have any side effects or difficulty sleeping, you should also let your doctor know. They may be able to adjust your medication or recommend other therapies for you, like melatonin, a hormone that controls your sleep cycle, or a CPAP machine, a machine that improves breathing while you sleep.

- Maintain proper sleep hygiene and abstain from actions that might interfere with your sleep or make it more difficult to fall asleep. Taking a nap during the day might cause you to feel less drowsy at night, therefore you should avoid doing so. A lot of fluid consumption right before bed might also cause you to wake up needing to urinate. Additionally, you should try to avoid staring at the clock since it may aggravate or frighten you. Additionally, you should refrain from monitoring your computer, tablet, or phone since they release blue light, which might inhibit your melatonin synthesis or keep you awake.

You may live well with Parkinson's disease and enhance your physical, mental, and emotional well-being by getting enough sleep.

Chapter Six

Addressing the emotional impact of a Parkinson's diagnosis

Receiving a Parkinson's disease diagnosis might come as a shock. You can experience fear, rage, sadness, or confusion. How this will impact your life, your family, and your future may be on your mind. You might not know where to look for assistance and you could have a lot of questions and worries. These are typical responses, and you're not the only one who experiences them.

Recognising your emotions and giving yourself permission to express them is the first step. You can speak with your physician, therapist, friends, family, or support group. In addition, you can journal, paint, draw, or enjoy some music. You can hit a pillow, yell, or cry. Whatever allows you to feel better and let go of your feelings.

Become knowledgeable about Parkinson's disease and what it implies for you is the second thing you should do. You can read trustworthy and current sources of information regarding the illness through books, articles, or websites. Additionally, you may view webinars, podcasts, and films featuring professionals and individuals who have Parkinson's disease. Additionally, you may go to conferences, seminars, and workshops that provide guidance and assistance. You can also discuss any questions or concerns you may have to your physician, therapist, or support group.

The third step is to focus on the things that you can influence and alter and to develop an optimistic and hopeful mindset. You may celebrate your successes and create reasonable, doable objectives. You may follow your passions, hobbies, or goals and discover meaning and purpose in your life. With your bravery and tenacity, you can also change the world and motivate others.

You may manage the stress, worry, and loss that come with receiving a Parkinson's diagnosis by attending to the emotional effect of the news. Additionally, you can raise your quality of life, mood, and self-esteem. Additionally, you can get ready for the chances and difficulties that lie ahead.

How to cope with anxiety, depression, and stress.

These typical Parkinson's disease non-motor symptoms can have an impact on your quality of life, happiness, and overall well-being. You may, however, learn coping mechanisms to enhance your emotional and mental well-being. I'll share some coping mechanisms with you in this area for stress, anxiety, and depression.

How to handle anxiety

Anxiety is a state of unease, concern, or terror that obstructs day-to-day functioning. Your symptoms, your future, your family, or your job might be causing you anxiety. Physical symptoms including sweating, shaking, a beating heart, or shortness of breath are also possible. You may avoid particular circumstances due to anxiety, or you may experience restlessness, irritability, or overload.

The following advice can help you manage your anxiety:

Determine the cause of your concern and confront your pessimistic ideas. You can pinpoint what causes your anxiety as well as your ideas and beliefs about it by using a notebook, worksheet, or app. Additionally, you can apply cognitive-behavioural therapy (CBT) strategies, which include questioning, reframing, and substituting more realistic or positive ideas for your negative ones. Other affirmations that you might use include "I can handle this," "I am not alone," and "This too shall pass."

Use methods of relaxation like mindfulness, meditation, or deep breathing. These can assist you in lowering your anxiety and calming your body and mind. You can practice these methods with the aid of a manual, a video, or an app. Additionally, aromatherapy using plants like rose, chamomile, or lavender might help you unwind. You can unwind with the aid of art, music, and the outdoors.

Talk to someone you can trust and look for social assistance. You can speak with your physician, therapist, friends, family, or support group. Anxiety and Depression

Association of America Helpline (https://adaa.org/finding-help/getting-support/support-groups) and the National Parkinson Foundation Helpline (https://www.parkinson.org/Living-with-Parkinsons/Resources-and-Support/Helpline) are two examples of helplines you may contact. You may express your emotions, gain guidance, and feel less alone by having a conversation with someone.

Seek expert assistance and think about taking medicine or treatment. You might need to contact a doctor or therapist if your anxiety is severe, ongoing, or interfering with your day-to-day activities. They can provide you treatment or medication and assist in diagnosing your anxiety. Although medicine may have negative effects or interfere with your Parkinson's medication, it might help you feel less anxious. You can learn skills and coping mechanisms to deal with your anxiety in therapy, which can help you understand and manage it. To assist you manage your anxiety, you can also try various therapies like acupuncture, biofeedback, or hypnosis.

You may enhance your quality of life, happiness, and wellbeing by learning coping mechanisms for anxiety. It's also possible to feel calmer, more in control, and more confident.

How to handle depression

Depression is characterised by a lingering sense of hopelessness, unhappiness, or disinterest in activities you used to like. Your symptoms, diagnosis, life, or future plans might be the source of your depression. Physical symptoms including weariness, sleeplessness, changes in appetite, or changes in weight are also possible. Depression can cause social disengagement, motivation decline, and suicidal thoughts.

The following advice can help you deal with depression:

Acknowledge the symptoms of depression and get support. To evaluate your depression, you can utilise a screening instrument like the Patient Health Questionnaire (PHQ-9) (https://www.mdcalc.com/phq-9-patient-health-questionnaire-9). You may also keep an eye on your mood by using a mood tracker, which might be an app, a chart, or a journal. If your depressive symptoms last longer than two weeks or if you have thoughts of hurting yourself or other people, you should get treatment. You can speak with your physician, therapist, friends, family, or support group.

Another option is to give a call to a hotline, such the

National Parkinson Foundation Helpline

(https://www.parkinson.org/Living-with-

Parkinsons/Resources-and-Support/Helpline)   or   the

National   Suicide   Prevention   Lifeline

(https://suicidepreventionlifeline.org/).

**Seek expert assistance and think about taking medicine

or treatment.** You might need to consult a physician or

therapist if your depression is severe, ongoing, or causing

problems in your day-to-day activities. They can offer

treatment or medication and assist in diagnosing your

depression. Although medicine may have negative effects or

interfere with your Parkinson's medication, it can also help

you feel better. Counselling can teach you coping

mechanisms and help you comprehend and manage your

depression. To assist you deal with your depression, you can also try various therapies including deep brain stimulation (DBS), transcranial magnetic stimulation (TMS), or electroconvulsive therapy (ECT).

Take care of yourself and pursue your happiness. You may maintain your physical well-being by regular exercise, a healthy diet, and adequate sleep. Additionally, you may nurture your mental and emotional well-being by unwinding, practicing meditation, or engaging in creative endeavours. You can also pursue your interests, hobbies, or dreams—activities that bring you joy. You can also engage in positive activities like volunteering, giving to charity, and helping others. Another way to treat oneself is to spoil yourself, indulge yourself, or go overboard.

Reach out to people and establish connections. You can speak with your physician, therapist, friends, family, or support group. Additionally, you can participate in programs, clubs, and groups catered to individuals with Parkinson's disease. Examples of these include Parkinson's Movement Initiative (PMI) [https://www.americandancefestival.org/education/parkinsons-movement-initiative/], Parkinson's Wellness Recovery (PWR!) [https://www.pwr4life.org/]. You might feel less alone, more understood, and more supported when you connect with people.

You may raise your quality of life, your mood, and your overall wellbeing by learning coping mechanisms for depression. You may also experience an increase in optimism, fulfilment, and hope.

How to handle tension

Stress is the body's or mind's reaction to a demanding or dangerous circumstance. Your symptoms, diagnosis, life, or future plans might be causing you stress. Physical symptoms including headaches, stomachaches, or chest discomfort are also possible. Anxiety, depression, and rage are all possible reactions to stress. It may also have an impact on your heart, blood pressure, or immune system.

The following advice will help you manage stress:

Determine the cause of your stress and make an effort to lessen or get rid of it. You may track your stressors and your responses to them by keeping a diary, using a worksheet, or using an app. To assist you manage your stress, you may also employ problem-solving strategies like brainstorming, assessing, or putting solutions into practice. In order to manage your stress, you may also employ assertiveness techniques like saying no, establishing boundaries, and asking for assistance.

Use methods of relaxation like mindfulness, meditation, or deep breathing. These can assist you in lowering your stress level and calming your body and mind. You can practice these methods with the aid of a manual, a video, or an app. Additionally, aromatherapy using plants like rose, chamomile, or lavender might help you unwind. You can unwind with the aid of art, music, and the outdoors.

Talk to someone you can trust and look for social assistance. You can speak with your physician, therapist, friends, family, or support group. Alternatively, you can give a call to a hotline run by organisations like the Stress Management Society

For stress support: https://www.mentalhealth.gov/get-help/immediate-help

For Parkinson's support: https://www.parkinson.org/Living-with-Parkinsons/Resources-and-Support/helpline

You can seek advice, express your emotions, and feel less alone by talking to someone.

Seek expert assistance and think about taking medicine or treatment. You might need to contact a doctor or therapist if your stress is severe, ongoing, or interfering with your day-to-day activities. They can provide you treatment or medicines and assist in diagnosing your stress. Although medicine might help you feel less stressed, there is a chance that it can interfere with your Parkinson's medication or cause negative effects. Counselling may teach you coping mechanisms and help you understand and manage your stress. To assist you manage your stress, you can also try various therapies like acupuncture, biofeedback, or hypnosis.

You may raise your quality of life, your mood, and your overall wellbeing by learning how to manage stress. A sense of calmness, relaxation, and control may also increase.

How to Seek Professional Support and Counselling Services

A crucial component of your Parkinson's disease treatment and care is receiving professional support and counselling services. They can support you in overcoming the emotional, mental, and physical difficulties associated with having the illness. They can also assist you in enhancing your life's quality, health, and wellbeing. Physicians, therapists, counsellors, psychologists, psychiatrists, social workers, and other health professionals are examples of professionals who provide professional assistance and counselling services. They can diagnose you and treat you using medicine, treatment, counselling, education, and direction. Additionally, they can direct you to additional services and information that could be helpful.

Finding, selecting, and utilizing professional support and counseling services are the three steps involved in the process.

Locate: It might be difficult, but not impossible, to find a trained and experienced specialist who can assist you with your unique needs and preferences. To locate a specialist, you can utilise a variety of resources and techniques, including: Requesting a reference or suggestion from your family physician, neurologist, or movement disorder specialist. They could know someone with expertise treating patients with Parkinson's disease or who specialises in the condition.

Requesting a reference or referral from your friends, family, or support network. They could know someone who has, or they might have worked with someone they trust in the past.

Looking for experts that provide Parkinson's disease support and counselling services online or through directories, databases, or websites. The [National Association of Social Workers (NASW) Find a Social Worker] (https://www.socialworkers.org/online-directory), the [American Psychological Association (APA) Psychologist Locator] (https://locator.apa.org/), and the [Parkinson's Foundation Helpline] (https://www.parkinson.org/Living-with-Parkinsons/Resources-and-Support/Helpline) are a few examples.

Making contact with regional or national Parkinson's disease organizations, such as the World Parkinson Coalition, the Michael J. Fox Foundation, or the Parkinson's Foundation.

They could provide support and counseling services directly, or they might provide programs, tools, or information that might assist you in finding a professional.

Select: Selecting a professional that can fulfill your objectives and expectations might be challenging, but it's not impossible. To select a professional, you might consider a variety of elements and criteria, including:

Qualifications and credentials: Verify the validity and timeliness of the professional's degrees, training, certificates, and licenses. Additionally, you should confirm that the professional's experience, knowledge, and area of specialization are appropriate and meet your demands.

Availability and accessibility: Make sure the professional is convenient and within your budget by looking up their location, hours, and rates. Additionally, you should confirm with the expert that they can meet you at your convenience or within an acceptable amount of time by checking their availability. Additionally, you should confirm that the expert is reachable and that they can converse with you in the language, format, or mode that you choose.

Compatibility and rapport: See how you feel about the expert after an in-person meeting, phone consultation, or video consultation. It might be beneficial to pose questions to them and observe their responses. Seek out a professional who is kind, understanding, and encouraging. Additionally, you want to search for a professional that exudes confidence, competence, and expertise. Additionally, you want to search for a professional that shares your ideals, style, and attitude. Additionally, you want to search for a professional that can get along well with you and make you feel at ease and reliable.

Use: Getting support and counseling from a professional might be helpful, but it's not always simple. To employ the services of a professional, you can employ a variety of techniques and advice, including:

Make the most of your appointments by being prepared. One way to get ready is to write down any symptoms, worries, inquiries, or objectives and bring them with you to your sessions. Additionally, you are welcome to bring any pertinent paperwork, including your prescription list, test results, and medical records. If necessary or desired, you are welcome to bring additional family members, friends, or supporters. Making the most of your appointments may be achieved via cooperation, openness, and honesty. You may also be involved, inquiring, and proactive. You can also seek help, comments, or clarification. If necessary or desired, you may also jot down notes or record your appointments.

Assess and track your development and contentment. By establishing and assessing your objectives and tracking your results, you can assess and keep an eye on things. You can score your progress and satisfaction using a scale, a questionnaire, or a feedback form. You can also keep a log, a tracker, or a journal to document your activities, emotions, and symptoms. You may also keep an eye on your mood by using a mood tracker, which might be an app, a chart, or a journal. It is advisable that you periodically assess and track your accomplishments and contentment, then communicate them to your experts. Additionally, talk about any adjustments or issues you may be having to figure out how to deal with them.

Engage in dialogue and teamwork with your experts. By staying in contact with your specialists and providing them with updates on your position, you can foster collaboration and communication. You can also adhere to their recommendations and complete your treatment or take your medicine as directed. Additionally, you may appreciate their knowledge and ask for their advice. Respect your experience and feel free to express your opinions as well. Respecting and expressing your emotions are other options. Additionally, you may respect one another's opinions and offer and accept comments. Along with cooperating, you may respect one another's duties.

You may live well with Parkinson's disease and enhance your physical, mental, and emotional well-being by obtaining expert assistance and counseling services. You may also experience more empowerment, understanding, and support.

Chapter Seven

BUILDING A SUPPORT NETWORK

It might be difficult to live with Parkinson's disease, but you don't have to do it by yourself. Your quality of life, health, and well-being may all be significantly improved by surrounding yourself with kind and understanding individuals. A support system can help you manage the psychological, practical, and emotional elements of the illness by offering you emotional, practical, and informational assistance. A support system may also help you enjoy life and find new things to love, as well as keep you engaged, optimistic, and connected.

Anyone who is encouraging, reliable, and compassionate, such as friends, family, medical professionals, support organisations, and other Parkinson's disease sufferers, can be a part of your support network. Additionally, you may increase the size of your support system by contacting groups that specialise in Parkinson's disease, the local community, and internet resources. But creating and sustaining a support system can be difficult, particularly if you live alone, have limited mobility, or experience prejudice or stigma. You must thus be proactive, adaptable, and resourceful in locating and obtaining the assistance you require.

The value of assistance from friends, family, and medical professionals

Professionals in the medical field, friends, and family are frequently the mainstays of your support system. They are able to provide you several forms of assistance, including:

Support that makes you feel loved, cared for, and understood is known as emotional support. It can involve showing affection, consoling, encouraging, or listening. You may manage stress, anxiety, despair, and loneliness with the aid of emotional support. Additionally, it can boost your resilience, resilience, and mood.

Support that is helpful with day-to-day duties and activities is known as practical support. It can involve completing tasks for you, such as driving, shopping, cooking, cleaning, or tending to your pets. You may preserve your freedom, functionality, and performance with the aid of practical support. Additionally, it can assist you in avoiding or lessening consequences like injuries, illnesses, or falls.

Support that is informational: This kind of assistance aids in your comprehension and awareness of Parkinson's disease. It might involve giving, receiving, or requesting information in the form of data, guidelines, recommendations, or sources. You can control your disease, make educated decisions, and educate yourself with the use of informational support. It may also make it easier for you to take advantage of additional possibilities or services.

Different forms of support can be offered by your family, friends, and healthcare professionals based on their responsibilities, connections, and areas of competence. As an illustration:

Since your family is often the closest and most involved in your life, they may offer you both practical and emotional support. They may have studied Parkinson's disease independently or with you, so they may also provide you informative assistance.

Since your friends are usually the ones who share your interests, passions, and hobbies, they may provide you both practical and emotional support. They can also provide you informative assistance since they could share your experiences, difficulties, or objectives, or they might know people who can assist you.

**Your healthcare providers are frequently the most knowledgeable, skilled, and experienced in treating and caring for Parkinson's disease, so they can offer you

both practical and informative help. Because they could appreciate, empathize with, and have empathy for you and your situation, they might also offer you emotional support.

You may enhance your quality of life, health, and well-being by seeking help from friends, family, and medical experts. You may also experience more empowerment, understanding, and support.

How to get in touch with neighborhood services and support organizations.

These are associations or groups that provide advocacy, education, and support to individuals and families dealing with Parkinson's disease. They can assist you in connecting with others who share your objectives, struggles, and experiences. They can also assist you in getting access to opportunities, services, or information that might be helpful.

You can take the following actions to get in touch with neighbourhood services and support groups:

1. Look for local Parkinson's disease support groups and resources on the internet by using directories, websites, or databases. The American Parkinson Disease Association (APDA) Local Resources (https://www.apdaparkinson.org/community/), the Parkinson's Foundation Local Resources (https://www.parkinson.org/Living-with-Parkinsons/Resources-and-Support/Local-Resources), are a few examples.

2. Make contact with regional or national Parkinson's disease organisations, such as the World Parkinson Coalition, the Michael J. Fox Foundation, or the

Parkinson's Foundation. They could provide support groups or services themselves, or they might have programs, resources, or information that might help you locate one in your region.

3. Request recommendations or referrals from your loved ones, medical professionals, or other acquaintances. They could be aware of a resource or support group that they have personally utilised, heard about, or know someone who has.

4. Check to determine whether the resource or support group you are interested in meets your requirements and preferences by giving them a call or visiting. You are welcome to enquire about their services, policies, clientele, meeting schedule, location, hours, and price. Additionally, you may offer them a sample or a trial,

like going to a meeting, getting a newsletter, or using a service.

5. Make the most of the resource or support group you choose by joining or using it. You are welcome to take part in their social events, workshops, lectures, and meetings. Their services, which include advocacy, education, and counselling, might also be advantageous to you. Additionally, you may support their community by lending your voice, your experience, or your narrative. To assist them in developing or growing, you may also offer money, recommendations, or comments.

6. You may enhance your quality of life, health, and well-being by making connections with neighbourhood services and support organisations.

It's also possible to feel positive, involved, and more connected. You can also find new things to love and enjoy life.

Tips for communicating with loved ones about Parkinson's disease.

Sharing your needs, wants, and worries with your loved ones might help you both feel better. It can also assist you in obtaining empathy, comprehension, and support. In addition, it may make your time together more enjoyable and help you preserve and build your connections.

But talking to your loved ones about your Parkinson's disease can sometimes be challenging, particularly if you're not used to discussing your concerns, feelings, or health. Barriers like fear, denial, guilt, or humiliation might also be present. It's also possible that your expectations, tastes, and communication styles differ. As a result, when speaking with your loved ones, you should be truthful, forthright, and courteous. You may also use some tricks and techniques to make the process go more smoothly.

How to disclose your diagnosis to your loved ones

One of the most difficult, yet equally crucial, things to do is to inform your loved ones of your illness. It can support you in overcoming any shock, tension, or grief you may encounter. Additionally, it might assist you in obtaining the empathy, comprehension, and support you want. Additionally, it might assist you in preparing yd do our friends and family for any upcoming changes and difficulties.

However, it may also be unsettling, distressing, or awkward to inform your loved ones about your diagnosis. You could be at a loss for words or how to strike up a discussion. It's also possible that you have no idea what to expect or how they will respond. You can also be concerned about bothering or disturbing them. As a result, to make things simpler and more efficient, prepare ahead of time and employ some tricks and techniques.

The following advice will help you inform your loved ones and friends about your diagnosis:

Select the ideal time and location. It is important that you and your loved ones pick a convenient, private, and comfortable time and location. Additionally, pick a time and location that will provide you adequate space, time, and focus to conduct the talk. Telling them while you're pressed for time, in public, or under pressure is not something you should do.

Get ready to express what you want to. It is advisable that you prepare your thoughts and delivery. Additionally, you should decide how much and what you want to disclose.

You may organize your ideas and words by using an outline, a script, or a note. Additionally, you can rehearse your speech on your own or with a reliable person.

Be forthright and truthful. Regarding your diagnosis and its implications for you, you ought to be forthright and honest. It's also important to be open and explicit about your needs, wants, and worries. Avoid using euphemisms or jargon and stick to plain, straightforward English instead. In order to strengthen your arguments and humanise them, you should also use anecdotes or instances. Along with responding to their inquiries, you ought to point them in the direction of further resources of knowledge, like your therapist, doctor, or support group.

Be upbeat and optimistic. Regarding your diagnosis and what it implies for you, you should have optimism and hope.

You ought to have optimism and hope for your life and the future. The benefits of your disease, such as the therapies, treatments, and support systems at your disposal, should be highlighted. It is also important to highlight the good parts of your life, such your aspirations, ambitions, and hobbies. Additionally, you ought to let people know how appreciative, upbeat, and resilient you are, and that Parkinson's illness does not define who you are.

Act with decency and compassion. Regarding the feelings and significance of your friends' and family's emotions, you have to show them respect and empathy. Additionally, you have to be considerate of their requirements, wants, and worries. You ought to respect their feelings and give credence to what they have gone through. Additionally, you ought to pay attention to what they have to say and value their viewpoints. You have to demonstrate your concern for them by lending them your support, empathy, and comprehension.

Informing your loved ones about your illness can help you live a better, healthier, and more fulfilling life. You may also experience more empowerment, understanding, and support.

How to ask for and accept help from your loved ones.

Getting support from your loved ones when you need it can help you manage the emotional, mental, and physical elements of the illness. It may also support you in preserving your autonomy, functionality, and output. Additionally, it can assist you in avoiding or lessening consequences like injuries, illnesses, or falls.

But it can also be difficult to ask for and accept assistance from your loved ones, particularly if you are accustomed to being proud, independent, or self-sufficient. Obstacles like fear, guilt, or humiliation could also arise. It's also possible that your requirements, tastes, or expectations differ. In order to make asking for and accepting assistance from your loved ones simpler and more successful, you should do it in an honest, courteous, and open manner. You may also utilise some helpful advice and techniques.

The following advice can help you both ask and accept assistance from your loved ones:

Determine your tastes and needs. Prioritise your requirements and preferences based on their urgency and significance after you have identified them. Along with identifying your abilities and limitations, you should also note what you need assistance with. You may arrange your requirements and preferences with the use of an app, chart, or list. To score your requirements and preferences, you may alternatively use a scale, a questionnaire, or a feedback form.

Express your choices and demands. It's important to let others know what you need and prefer, why you need support, and how you'd like to get it. Additionally, you should gently and clearly state your requirements, wants, and concerns. It is best to speak simply and directly; do not criticise, demand, or place blame. In order to strengthen your arguments and humanise them, you should also use anecdotes or instances. It's important to respect your loved ones' viewpoints and pay attention to what they have to say.

Request precise and practical assistance. It is best to be particular and reasonable in your demands for assistance rather than general or exaggerated. Additionally, you ought to request assistance from your loved ones that fits your tastes and demands. Additionally, you should allow your loved ones adequate time, space, and attention to assist you and ask for aid in advance. Additionally, you have to request assistance in a courteous manner by using phrases like "please," "thank you," or "I appreciate."

Accept assistance with gratitude and grace. It is best to accept assistance with gratitude and grace rather than to reject, refuse, or voice complaints. Additionally, you ought to take assistance from your loved ones that fits your preferences and demands. Additionally, you ought to view assistance as a gift rather than a liability, debt, or favour. Additionally, when accepting assistance, put on a grin and say something like "thank you," "I appreciate," or "you're amazing."

I truly and freely return the favour by helping you. Help should be freely and truly returned; do not ignore, neglect, or take assistance for granted. Help that fits your loved ones' requirements and preferences and that you are able to offer should be returned. Additionally, you ought to return favours as a gesture rather than as a duty, obligation, or remuneration. When offering assistance, remember to smile and say something like "you're welcome," "I'm happy to help," or "you're awesome."

You may enhance your quality of life, health, and well-being by seeking and receiving assistance from your loved ones. You may also experience more empowerment, understanding, and support.

Chapter Eight

PLANNING FOR THE FUTURE

The disorder known as Parkinson's disease impairs both your motor and cognitive abilities. It results from the death or malfunction of some of the brain cells that produce the neurotransmitter dopamine. Your brain uses dopamine to regulate both your emotions and your muscles. Reduced dopamine levels can cause issues with mood, balance, stiffness, slowness, and tremors.

Parkinson's disease can have an impact on your life as well as your health. It may have an impact on your future, family, career, and income. It may also have an impact on your decisions, inclinations, and desires. As a result, it is critical to make plans for the future and get ready for any obstacles or changes that may arise. You may take charge of your life and assist yourself and your loved ones deal with the disease by making plans for the future. Making plans for the future can also help you enjoy life, find new interests, and manage your Parkinson's disease properly.

Discussing long-term considerations, such as financial planning and legal matters

Parkinson's disease may significantly affect your rights and obligations under the law, as well as your financial status. You could have to pay more for long-term care, home improvements, or medical bills. Reduced income might also be an issue for you if you're unemployed, retired, or disabled. Legal matters including powers of attorney, trusts, and wills might also come up. It is crucial to talk about and prepare for these long-term issues as a result. You can safeguard your finances, preserve your possessions, and make sure your intentions are carried out by having a conversation about these long-term issues. Talking about these long-term issues might also help you steer clear of future tension, misunderstanding, or conflict.

The following advice can be used when talking about long-term issues like financial planning and legal issues:

Seek competent counsel and assistance from professionals. You ought to have competent counsel and meet with specialists that can assist you with legal and financial preparation. Financial planners, accountants, attorneys, and social workers are a few examples of these specialists. They can provide you advice on the finest alternatives and approaches for your requirements and objectives as well as assist you in evaluating your present and future financial status. They may also assist you with updating and preparing your legal documentation and serve as your advocate in court. These professionals can be located by recommendations, referrals, or online directories like the National Association of Social Workers (NASW) (https://www.socialworkers.org/online-directory), the American Institute of Certified Public Accountants (AICPA) (https://www.aicpa.org/forthepublic/findacpa.html), the American Bar Association (ABA) (https://www.americanbar.org/groups/legal_services/flh-home/), or the Financial Planning Association (FPA) (https://www.plannersearch.org/).

Engage your loved ones and maintain communication with them. It is advisable to consult with your loved ones and friends on legal issues and financial preparedness. They might be able to support you in your actions or offer advice on decisions you make. They could also play a part in or be impacted by your legal and financial preparation. As a result, you have to enlighten them and pay attention to their thoughts and worries. In addition, you have to be considerate of their choices and feelings while working toward a compromise or consensus. Additionally, you ought to let them know how much you value and appreciate them.

Maintain organization in your plans and documentation by reviewing and updating them. Plans and documentation should be reviewed and updated, and they should be kept organized and easily available. Your health, income, costs, ambitions, and legal difficulties are all subject to change over time, and this might have an impact on your financial status and legal issues. As a result, you should constantly evaluate and update your plans and documentation to ensure that they accurately reflect your requirements and preferences both now and in the future. It is advisable to have your plans and records well-organized, easily accessible, and stored in a secure location.

Additionally, you have to duplicate your ideas and paperwork and provide them to dependable buddies, family members, or experts.

You may enhance your quality of life and general health by talking about long-term issues including financial planning and legal issues. You may experience an increase in readiness, self-assurance, and mastery.

The significance of recording healthcare choices and engaging in advance care planning.

While it might be a delicate subject, Parkinson's disease patients and their families need to know about it. The process of organising your future medical care in the event that you are unable to make or express decisions for yourself is known as advance care planning. You may save your desires, morals, and aspirations for your medical treatment in case you need to refer to them later by documenting your healthcare preferences. You may make sure that your healthcare is provided in accordance with your wants and that your family and healthcare professionals are aware of your choices by completing advance care planning and recording your healthcare preferences.

The following advice will help you record your healthcare preferences and prepare for future care:

Commence early and provide frequent updates. As soon as possible, you should begin creating an advance care plan and recording your healthcare choices. You should also update these documents on a regular basis or whenever your preferences, circumstances, or health change. In order to ensure that your family and medical professionals are aware of and respect them, you should also go over them with them.

Select a backup plan and a health care proxy. If you are unable to make choices for yourself regarding your health, someone else can act as your health care proxy. Someone who can take over in the event that your health care proxy is unable or unwilling is known as a backup. Selecting a backup and a health care proxy who are dependable, trustworthy, and prepared to act on your behalf is advised. Additionally, you want to pick someone who is well-versed in your desires and has the ability to express them. Additionally, you want to pick someone who is easily reachable or who lives nearby. Additionally, you should provide copies of your records to your backup and health care proxy, as well as explain to them their duties.

Finish writing a living will and an advance directive. A formal document known as an advance directive outlines your backup plan and health care proxy. Your healthcare choices, including the kinds of treatments you desire or don't want and the quality of life you value or don't value, can be expressed in a living will, a legal document. You should abide with your state's rules and regulations and write an advance directive and a living will that are legitimate and recognised in your state. If you want assistance or direction, you should also speak with your physician, attorney, or social worker. In addition, if your state requires it, you should get your documents witnessed and notarised in addition to signing and dating them.

Save and distribute your files and preferences. Your papers and preferences should be shared and stored, and you should make sure they are easily accessible in case you need them. Your records and preferences should be kept in a secure location, such an online register, a safe deposit box, or a fireproof box. It is advisable to provide your documentation and choices to your relatives, backup, health care proxy, physicians, and any other individuals who could be engaged in your medical care. Additionally, you have to keep a card, bracelet, or sticker on you at all times that states where your living will and advance directive are located.

You may enhance your quality of life, well-being, and physical and mental health by proactively planning and recording your healthcare choices. You may experience an increase in readiness, self-assurance, and mastery.

Resources for navigating insurance coverage and disability benefits

Your insurance coverage and access to disability benefits, as well as your eligibility for them, may be significantly impacted by Parkinson's disease. It might be difficult for you to obtain sufficient and reasonably priced insurance, to apply for and be granted disability benefits, or to appeal or renew your claims. As a result, it's critical that you understand your options and rights and make use of the tools available to assist you in navigating the insurance and disability systems. You may safeguard your quality of life, your money, and your health by using these resources.

The following resources can help you understand disability compensation and insurance coverage:

For those with Parkinson's disease and their families, the Parkinson's Foundation Insurance and Financial Assistance website (https://www.parkinson.org/Living-with-Parkinsons/Insurance-and-Financial-Assistance) offers resources, advice, and connections to a number of insurance and financial assistance programs and services. Financial planning, prescription medication assistance, long-term care insurance, Medicare, Medicaid, and private insurance are among the subjects it addresses.

For those with Parkinson's disease and their families, the [American Parkinson Disease Association (APDA)] Disability Benefits website

(https://www.apdaparkinson.org/resources-support/disability-benefits/) offers information, advice, and links to a number of disability benefits programs and services. It addresses issues including workers' compensation, veterans benefits, Supplemental Security Income (SSI), and Social Security Disability Insurance (SSDI).

The [Parkinson's Foundation Helpline]

(https://www.parkinson.org/Living-with-Parkinsons/Resources-and-Support/Helpline) is a toll-free number that puts you in contact with a qualified staff member who can respond to your inquiries, offer advice, and direct you to additional services and resources that might be of assistance. The hotline may be reached by phone from 9 a.m. to 8 p.m. ET, Monday through Friday, at 1-800-4PD-INFO (473-4636).

You can get free legal advice and assistance on matters related to Parkinson's disease, such as insurance, disability, employment, or estate planning, by visiting the Parkinson's Foundation Legal Clinic

(https://www.parkinson.org/Living-with-Parkinsons/Resources-and-Support/Legal-Clinic).

By completing an online form or giving the hotline a call at 1-800-4PD-INFO (473-4636), you may make a consultation request.

You may enhance your quality of life, health, and wellbeing by making use of these resources. You may also experience more empowerment, understanding, and support.

Chapter Nine

STAYING INFORMED AND EMPOWERED

Even though living with Parkinson's disease might be difficult, you don't have to give up on your hobbies, objectives, or goals. If you remain knowledgeable and in control of your life, you may still have a happy and meaningful one.

Promoting self-advocacy and active involvement in treatment choices

Being an active participant in your treatment decisions and an advocate for yourself is one of the most essential things you can do as a person with Parkinson's disease. This implies that you:

- Talk honestly and freely about your objectives, preferences, worries, and symptoms with your healthcare staff.

- If anything confuses or unnerves you, ask questions and get explanation.

- Learn as much as you can about your illness, available treatments, and any possible adverse effects.

- Respect other people's thoughts and preferences while expressing your own.

- If you are uncomfortable or dissatisfied with your present course of therapy, get a second opinion.

- Include your friends, family, and support system in the choices you make about your care.

- Honor your right to secrecy and privacy.

Being an active participant in your treatment decisions and a self-advocate allows you to:

- Boost your happiness and quality of life with your care.

- Boost your trust and rapport with your medical staff.

- Become more empowered and in charge of your life.

- Lessen your worry and tension.

- Improve results and steer clear of needless difficulties.

Keeping up with developments and research on Parkinson's

Parkinson's disease is a progressive, multifaceted illness that affects individuals differently. Parkinson's disease does not have a cure, but there are several therapies and treatments that can help control the symptoms and enhance quality of life. However, new advancements and discoveries are being made daily in the field of Parkinson's research, which is always changing and growing. As a result, it's critical to keep up with the most recent findings and innovations in Parkinson's disease research.

This can assist you:

- Find out about cutting-edge therapies and treatments that might help people with Parkinson's disease, including you.

- Recognise the advantages and disadvantages of taking part in research studies and clinical trials.

- Learn about the resources and support services, both current and new, that can help you manage your disease.

- Make connections with other Parkinson's disease sufferers who have similar interests and experiences.

- Encourage and assist organisations and the Parkinson's research community in their endeavours.

There are several ways to remain up to date on developments in Parkinson's disease research, including:

- Following blogs, podcasts, journals, social media channels, newsletters, and other publications that offer current and accurate information about Parkinson's disease

- Visiting reliable websites and online resources, such as the [Parkinson's Foundation] https://www.parkinson.org/). the [Michael J. Fox Foundation](https://www.michaeljfox.org/), the [Parkinson's US](https://www.parkinson.org/.), and the [World Parkinson

Coalition](https://www.worldpdcoalition.org/), that provide reliable and thorough information on Parkinson's disease.

.

- Participating in webinars, conferences, workshops, seminars, and other gatherings featuring leaders and specialists in the field of Parkinson's disease research and developments

- Getting involved in offline and online communities, networks, support groups, and forums that match you with other Parkinson disease sufferers who want to learn about and discuss Parkinson research and developments

- Speaking with your medical team, particularly your neurologist, about the most recent breakthroughs and prospects in Parkinson's disease research and development

Gaining the ability to govern your own health and wellbeing

Taking charge of your health and well-being is another essential component of remaining knowledgeable and in control.

This implies that you:

- Adhere to your specified regimen and take your drugs on time.

- Keep an eye on your symptoms and let your medical team know if anything changes or causes you worry.

- Keep up a nutritious, well-balanced diet that satisfies your tastes and nutritional requirements.

- Exercise and physical activity on a regular basis according to your capabilities and objectives.

- Make sure you get adequate rest and relaxation, and maintain excellent sleep hygiene.

- Handle your emotions and stress in a constructive and healthy manner.

- If you exhibit any indications of depression, anxiety, or other mental health problems, get professional assistance.

- Follow your passions, hobbies, and interests that make you happy and fulfilled.

- Maintain relationships with your loved ones, close friends, and support system.

- When you need assistance, ask for it and accept it.

Taking charge of your wellbeing and health allows you to:

- Boost your wellbeing on the mental, emotional, and physical levels.

- Lessen the severity and advancement of your problems and symptoms.

- Boost your confidence and sense of self-worth.

- Boost your ability to cope and be resilient.

- Have a more fulfilling and joyful existence.

Chapter Ten

Finding hope and support

Parkinson's disease does not have to limit who you are or what you can achieve. It may be a challenging and lonely illness. You still have the ability to express your optimism and support with other people.

Finding stories of resilience and hope from individuals living well with Parkinson's disease

Finding inspiration and encouragement from the experiences and tales of those who are successfully managing Parkinson's disease is one of the finest places to start. These are individuals who have dealt with the difficulties and uncertainties brought on by Parkinson's disease while also managing to adapt, prosper, and cope. These are individuals who have not allowed Parkinson's to stop them from following their objectives, hobbies, or passions. These are individuals who, in the face of hardship, have exhibited fortitude, bravery, and optimism. They are individuals with knowledge and inspiration to share with us.

There are several resources available for reading inspirational tales of resiliency and hope from people with Parkinson's disease, including:

Perusing written works by and about individuals with Parkinson's disease, including [Always Looking Up: The Adventures of an Incurable Optimist]Michael J. Fox's book Always Looking Up: Adventures Incurable (https://www.amazon.com/dp/1401310168)[A Woman's Guide to Parkinson's Disease: Parkinson's Diva][Perseverance: The Seven Skills You Need to Survive, Thrive, and Accomplish More Than You Ever Imagined] (https://www.amazon.com/Perseverance-Skills-Survive-

Accomplish-Imagined/dp/0735233666) by Tim Hague and Maria De Leon (https://www.amazon.com/Parkinsons-Diva-Womans-Guide-Disease/dp/149177099X) by Maria De Leon consuming podcasts, films, interviews, and documentaries with Parkinson's disease sufferers, including [Ride with Larry] (https://www.ridewithlarrymovie.com/), [When Life Gives You Parkinson's] (https://globalnews.ca/tag/when-life-gives-you-parkinsons/), and [The Michael J. Fox Show] (https://www.imdb.com/title/tt2338232/), as well as going to websites and online platforms like [Parkinson's Life] (https://parkinsonslife.eu/), [Davis Phinney Foundation] (https://davisphinneyfoundation.org/), and [Parkinson's Movement] (https://parkinsonsmovement.com/) that feature inspiring tales of resiliency and hope from people with Parkinson's.

Participating in Parkinson's disease celebrations and initiatives, such as Parkinson's Heroes (https://www.parkinson.org/get-involved.), World Parkinson's Day (https://www.worldpdcoalition.org/page/WPD), and Parkinson's Champions (https://www.parkinson.org/get-involved/Parkinsons-champions),

Finding inspiring and uplifting accounts from people who are effectively managing their Parkinson's disease will help you:

- Obtain understanding and perspective on your own state of affairs.

- Discover techniques and advice for handling your problems and symptoms.

- Find fresh, fascinating prospects and chances for your life.

- Feel inspired and driven to overcome your challenges and realise your objectives.

- Make a connection with and relate to those who are experiencing similar things as you.

- Recognise that there is a community of people that support and encourage you and that you are not alone.

Encouragement

Coping with the changes and restrictions that Parkinson's disease may bring about in your life is one of the challenges of having the condition. Sometimes you could feel helpless, depressed, furious, or frustrated. You could be concerned about your ability to continue doing the activities you enjoy or reach your own objectives. It's possible that you feel alone, misinterpreted, or unsupported by people.

But you shouldn't let Parkinson's disease prevent you from living life to the fullest and achieving your individual objectives. Parkinson's illness does not imply you have to give up on pleasure, meaning, or purpose in your life. You still have the ability to pursue your passions and take advantage of fresh, intriguing chances. You still have the ability to develop yourself, learn new things, and make a special contribution to the world.

In spite of Parkinson's disease, consider the following advice and ideas

for living life to the fullest and achieving your goals:

Consider your strengths rather than your weaknesses.
Parkinson's disease may have an impact on your capabilities, but it does not define you or what you are capable of. You still possess a wealth of abilities, skills, and capabilities that you may hone and utilise. You still have a lot of passions, interests, and pastimes to pursue. You still have a lot of ideas, aspirations, and ambitions that you may work toward and accomplish. Consider what you can do and do it well, rather than focusing on what you cannot.

Make significant and doable objectives for yourself.
Setting and achieving objectives may help you feel driven, accomplished, and have direction. But you must ensure that your objectives are both attainable and significant to you.

Achievable and quantifiable objectives that take into account your present circumstances and skills are considered realistic. Objectives that are in line with your beliefs, interests, and passions are considered meaningful. These are the objectives that are important to you and provide you a sense of fulfilment. Think about the following inquiries when you're establishing your own objectives: What do I desire to do? Why am I motivated to do it? How am I going to do that? How will I be able to tell whether I succeeded?

Divide your objectives into more doable, smaller steps. Your ambitions may occasionally appear too lofty or distant to achieve. You can feel overburdened, defeated, or irritated by this. You must divide your objectives into smaller, more doable tasks in order to prevent this. Every step you take to get closer to your objective should be precise and actionable. To help you feel like you're making progress and reaching your goals, every step you take should also be satisfying and doable. If your objective is to create a book, for instance, you may divide it up into manageable phases like selecting a subject, creating chapter summaries, composing the first draft, editing and rewriting, publishing, and advertising.

Ask for and accept support and assistance from others. It's not necessary for you to do everything alone. You can ask for and accept support and assistance from those who can help you reach your objectives. These might be your friends, family, medical staff, support system, mentor, coach, or anybody else who can provide you with direction, advice, criticism, encouragement, or support. You may gain from the knowledge, experience, and viewpoint of others by asking for and accepting their assistance and support. You may also boost your motivation and confidence while lowering your workload and stress levels. In addition, you'll feel more understood and supported as you develop and fortify your bonds with other people.

Honor your accomplishments and victories. It's difficult to pursue your own objectives and reach your ambitions, particularly if you have Parkinson's disease. Thus, regardless of how great or tiny your accomplishments are, you should be proud of them. You should be pleased with what you have accomplished and give yourself credit for your diligence and hard work. Along with rewarding yourself for your accomplishments, you ought to treat yourself to something enjoyable and meaningful. You may increase your pleasure and sense of self-worth by acknowledging and appreciating your accomplishments. Additionally, you may inspire yourself to persevere and reach new heights.

Resources for ongoing support and inspiration

Parkinson's disease might make it difficult to embrace life and pursue personal objectives, but you don't have to do it alone. There are many of resources available to offer you continuous encouragement and support. These tools can assist you in managing your symptoms, adjusting to your condition, enhancing your quality of life, and accomplishing your objectives.

You have access to the following tools:

Parkinson's Foundation: This national organization supports individuals with Parkinson's disease and their families by offering information, education, research, and advocacy. A few of the programs and services they provide are the following: [Parkinson's Advocacy Network (https://www.parkinson.org/get-involved/advocate), [PD Health @ Home (https://www.parkinson.org/pdhealth),

[Aware in Care] (https://www.parkinson.org/Living-with-Parkinsons/Resources-and-Support/Patient-Safety-Kit), and [Parkinson's Outcomes Project] (https://www.parkinson.org/research/Parkinsons-Outcomes-Project), and [Parkinson's Outcomes Project].

The Michael J. Fox Foundation is an international organization that provides funding and assistance for the advancement of efforts to discover a treatment for Parkinson's disease. Additionally, they offer services, education, and information to individuals with Parkinson's disease and their families. They provide a range of services and programs, including [Team Fox] (https://www.michaeljfox.org/teamfox), [Parkinson's 360] (https://www.michaeljfox.org/parkinsons-360), and [Fox Trial Finder] (https://foxtrialfinder.michaeljfox.org/).

Parkinson's US: People with Parkinson's disease and their families may get information, support, and research from this US-based organization. The organization provides a range of services and programs, including Parkinson's Online Forum (www.parkinson.org/community/forum.), Parkinson's Helpline (https://www.parkinson.org/Living-with-Parkinsons/Resources-and-Support/helpline.), Parkinson's Local Advisers (https://www.apdaparkinson.org/resources-support/), and Parkinson's Research Network (https://www.parkinson.org/research/Research-Advocates.).

The World Parkinson's Coalition is an international organization that unites people with Parkinson's disease worldwide to promote cooperation, dialogue, and education. They host the triennial [World Parkinson Congress] (https://www.worldpdcoalition.org/page/WPC2022), which

includes seminars, posters, exhibitions, and discussions

pertaining to science, clinical practice, and lived experience.

The WPC Blog

(https://www.worldpdcoalition.org/blogpost/1434450/WP

C-Blog), the WPC Podcast

(https://www.worldpdcoalition.org/page/WPCPodcast),

the WPC Webinars

 (https://www.worldpdcoalition.org/page/WPCWebinars),

and the WPC Virtual

(https://www.worldpdcoalition.org/page/WPCVirtual)   are

some of the programs and services they provide.

These are just a few of the tools available to you for

continuous encouragement and support. Depending on your

requirements and tastes, you may discover a plethora of

additional materials either offline or online. In order to share your experiences, thoughts, and tales with others, you may also build your own resources, such a blog, podcast, video, book, or diary. Additionally, you may serve as a resource by providing any Parkinson's disease sufferers who might be in need with your assistance, encouragement, and support. You have the power to improve both your own and other people's lives by generating and using resources.

Conclusion

We have travelled through the intricacies of Parkinson's disease in this thorough investigation, from comprehending its causes to overcoming the numerous obstacles it poses. We started our adventure by learning the basics of Parkinson's disease, including its origin, symptoms, and the vital significance of early detection and treatment.

As we went through the diagnostic process and dealt with the emotional fallout, we realised how important it is to provide people the information and resources they need to go through this crucial stage with fortitude and optimism. We discussed the complexities of managing symptoms, providing doable tactics for treating both motor and non-motor symptoms and stressing the significance of promptly obtaining medical advice.

We also looked at the wide range of accessible therapy choices, including non-pharmacological therapies, cutting-edge scientific developments, and pharmaceutical interventions. We emphasised the value of individualised care plans that provide special consideration to each patient's preferences and objectives, enabling them to actively participate in their recovery process.

We explored the art of living well with Parkinson's disease, going beyond simple care and providing advice on preserving quality of life, adjusting to changes, and adopting holistic approaches to health and wellbeing. We talked about the often-ignored area of non-motor symptoms, recognising the significant emotional toll that a Parkinson's diagnosis takes and providing coping mechanisms and support-seeking techniques.

The significance of creating a strong support system that includes friends, family, medical experts, and neighbourhood support groups was at the center of our conversation. We highlighted how connections and communities can develop resilience, empowerment, and a feeling of belonging.

As we looked ahead, we realised how important it was to make plans for the future—from advanced care planning and healthcare choices to financial and legal concerns. Our long-term goal is to reduce stress and anxiety by enabling people to take the initiative to initiate these conversations and successfully negotiate the intricacies of insurance coverage and disability compensation.

Let's reiterate the significance of remaining aware and in control, standing up for oneself, and facing life head-on as we come to the end of our trip together. The inspiring tales of tenacity and optimism that people with Parkinson's disease share with us serve as a constant reminder of the limitless opportunities that lay ahead of us, even in the face of obstacles.

Finally, keep in mind that your Parkinson's disease is just one chapter in the greater story of your life; it does not define you. You possess resiliency, strength, and the ability to triumph over hardship. Take guts, grit, and a firm confidence in your own value and embrace every day. Let's travel this road together with grace, resiliency, and unflinching optimism.

www.ingramcontent.com/pod-product-compliance
Lightning Source LLC
Chambersburg PA
CBHW051615250726

48653CB00004BA/1521